Brain Health

How to handle your head

by
Sharon Platt-McDonald
MSc RHV RM RGN

First published 2010

© 2010 The Stanborough Press Ltd

British Library Cataloguing in Publication Data.
A catalogue record for this book is available from the
British Library.

ISBN 1-904685-88-9

Published by The Stanborough Press Ltd,
Grantham, Lincolnshire.

Designed by Abigail Murphy

Printed in Thailand.

Introduction

The spotlight is on brain health. We look at what impacts brain development and degeneration, how to keep your brain healthy, how to boost memory and control the mind to enhance spiritual wellbeing.

We examine the factors that contribute to brain health and help prevent cognitive decline as we age. These are: dietary habits, physical activity, mental wellbeing and emotional stability, spirituality, social engagement and cardiovascular health.

Scientific discoveries have revealed new information about how the brain works and how we can use that knowledge to maximise brain health, particularly as we age.

When older adults challenge themselves with new thoughts and experiences, they not only create new neural pathways but they find new forms of self-expression. Research demonstrates the importance of developing new social and intellectual activities for the over 50s. This has been shown to halt the process of cognitive degeneration and enhance brain health well into the later stage of life.

Research tells us how to enhance the brain function of children and youth, the dangers and risks that can affect brain function at their particular age and its subsequent effect later in life.

Key principles

There is no greater or more complex system than the human brain. This collection of neurons weighing approximately 4 pounds initiates our thoughts, emotions and behaviour.

When we talk about staying fit, the general emphasis is from the neck down. However, the health of our brain plays a critical role in everything we do: thinking, feeling, remembering, working and playing – even sleeping.

You are what you eat

Two thirds of the brain is made up of fat. The food we eat provides building blocks to make these essential or 'good fats' called lipids which are crucial for effective brain function. However, 'bad fats' (trans fatty acids) can adversely affect the brain, causing difficulties from reduced learning ability to motor function difficulties and impaired mobility.

Use it or lose it

Although the brain is fully grown by age 6, activities such as reading, learning or processing information will cause new synapses to develop. Research suggests that an unchallenged or inactive mind may cause the number of synapses to decline. The number of synapses is closely linked with intelligence.

Play it smart

Avoid head injuries. Activities such as
cycling, equestrian sports and skating
have the potential for serious
accidents or damage to the brain.
Wearing a helmet can prevent this.
Studies on contact sports like soccer
have shown decreased cognitive skills
when repeated blows to the
head have occurred.

Drug alert

Many drugs have a damaging effect upon neurotransmitters, the chemicals which convey signals between nerve cells in the brain. Abusing drugs can kill brain cells.

Research indicates the following:

• The brain benefits from good nutrition and regular exercise.

• Environmental input such as aerobic exercise changes the structure and function of the brain.

• A proactive and lifelong lifestyle for brain health encourages the development of brain reserves that may delay the onset of neurodegenerative disease.

Chronic illness impact

Here we look at the impact of two long-term conditions on brain function.

Diabetes

• Diabetes damages the small blood vessels in the brain. This can eventually lead to those vessels closing off completely. When this occurs, the brain tissue fed by the blood vessel dies, causing a stroke.

• Several new research studies indicate that diabetes, and even pre-diabetes, damages brain cells directly.

• Recent research shows that people with diabetes are twice as likely to develop Alzheimer's disease.

If you are a diabetic it is crucial that you keep your blood sugars as normal and as tightly controlled as possible. New studies indicate that the better you control your blood sugars, the less brain damage you'll sustain. **Caution:** the higher the blood sugar levels, the more you harm your brain.

Advice

- Markedly reduce carbohydrate intake.

- Exercise and lead a more active lifestyle.

- Avoid saturated fats.

Hypertension

• Very high pressure can cause a break in a weakened blood vessel, which then bleeds in the brain. This can cause a stroke.

• A long-term study of 1,500 adults found that individuals with high cholesterol and high blood pressure had six times the risk of dementia.

Dr Louise Chang's research reviews the effects of hypertension on the brain. High blood pressure reduces blood flow to the area of the brain that controls memory and learning, perhaps raising the risk of Alzheimer's disease. *(WebMD Medical News.)*

Scans show that in people with Alzheimer's, blood flow to every part of the brain is substantially lower in those with hypertension.

Philip O. Alderson offers an explanation for this. Treated or not, high blood pressure makes the blood vessels narrower and less pliable over time. This hinders delivery of nutrients in the blood to the brain. 'Since Alzheimer's disease is marked by abnormal metabolism in an area of the brain associated with memory, poor delivery of nutrients to that part of the brain would make you more susceptible to the symptoms of Alzheimer's disease.'

Advice

- Monitor and control blood pressure.

- Reduce salt and saturated fats.

- Increase physical activity.

Physical wellbeing and the brain

You engage in exercise and healthy eating to maintain your physical health and wellbeing. But did you know that, in doing so, you are benefiting your mental health, too?

Studies highlight the mounting scientific evidence which shows that the positive lifestyle decisions you make now will help to reduce your risk of developing dementia later in life. Making the right changes in diet, exercise, mental stimulation and social interaction is not only good for you, but also good for your brain.

Researchers have found substantial evidence that with the optimal physical environment the brain continues to generate new brain cells throughout life. Studies indicated that challenging environments, which included a number of components such as learning opportunities, social interactions and physical activities, were key to boosting the growth of new brain cells.

Brain facts

• Oxygen plays a key role in brain health. Developing the efficiency and depth of your breathing improves brain function.

• Adequate water is essential to balancing physiological and biochemical processes in the body, as well as nerve and brain function.

• A diet rich in antioxidants slows the ageing process and diseases associated with brain degeneration.

- Exposure to toxic substances damages the brain, accelerates ageing and increases the incidence of memory loss.

- Unstable blood sugar levels damage brain cells and impair brain function.

- Thyroid dysfunction can impact mood and mental wellbeing.

- Exercise increases mental agility and alertness.

Nurture your body; nurture your brain and enhance its functional capacity.

Exercise impact

Today studies continue to demonstrate that exercise prevents the negative effects of chronic stress on the brain and boosts the brain's biological battle against infection.

Cell research shows that changes occur in the brain's learning and memory centre. Scientists are studying whether exercise alters the molecular mechanisms that are important for learning and memory.

An active lifestyle plays an important role in maintaining the function of the brain. Extensive research indicates the possibility that specialised exercise regimens may help repair damaged or aged brains.

Facts

Regular physical activity helps the blood flow to the brain. It also helps reduce the risk of heart attack, stroke and diabetes – all risk factors for dementia.

A recent study showed that people who exercised three or more times a week had a 30-40% lower risk of developing dementia than those who exercised fewer than three times a week. (*www.mentalhealth.org.uk*)

Exercising releases chemicals in the brain, like serotonin, that have a strong effect on mood, helping reduce anxiety, stress and depression.

Advice

The recommended level of physical activity is a minimum of 30 minutes of moderate activity most days of the week.

• Build up gradually if you're not used to being active. Sessions of 10-15 minutes 2-3 times a day is a good start and still produces results.

• Moderate activity includes brisk walking, strenuous gardening or jogging. This encourages good blood flow – enough to make you feel warmer and to increase heartbeat.

- Do activities that you enjoy.

- Go for regular walks or join a walking group.

- Instead of taking the car, walk or cycle, especially for short journeys.

- Get off the bus a stop or two earlier.

- Take the stairs instead of the lift when possible.

- Try something new like joining a gym, swimming or even dancing – at home!

Get moving!

The stress impact

Current research shows that stress can dramatically increase the ability of chemicals to pass through the blood-brain barrier (BBB). This became evident during the Gulf War, when soldiers experienced significant stress. The Israeli soldiers took a drug to protect themselves from chemical and biological weapons. Normally, it should not have crossed the BBB, but scientists learned that the stress of war had somehow increased the permeability of the BBB. Nearly one-quarter of the soldiers complained of headaches, nausea and dizziness – symptoms which occur only if the drug reaches the brain.

- A stress response is provoked by loud or sudden noises.

- Long-term over-secretion of stress hormones like cortisol adversely affects brain function, especially memory. Excess cortisol can prevent the brain from laying down new memory pathways, or from accessing already existing memories.

- Stress affects mental wellbeing and brain function. It can exacerbate a number of psychiatric disorders. A Yale University study looked at the effects of noise stress on brain function and found that stress impairs the cognitive function influencing dopamine, a key neurotransmitter that's involved in many brain disorders such as Parkinson's disease and even Attention Deficit Hyperactivity Disorder (ADHD).

- The level of noise at home or school affects children's ability to learn. Children living near airports or busy highways tend to have lower reading scores and develop language skills more slowly than children from quieter neighbourhoods.

- Chronic low-level noise affects brain and behaviour and has an insidious effect on health and wellbeing.

- Psychiatric hospitalisations are higher in noisy communities.

- Dr Alice H. Suter found that impaired learning, bad moods, aggression, lack of concentration, fatigue and poor work performance can result from continual exposure to the stress of unpleasant noise.

Advice

- Plan more 'quiet time' to enable you to pause and be still.

- In your quiet time ask God to fill you with his peace as you experience his presence.

- Relaxing in a calm environment allows you to de-stress, refresh your soul and replenish energy levels.

- Detox your mind by getting rid of negative thinking.

- Exercise daily.

- Get a prayer partner for support.

Nutrition and the brain

Researchers at the US Department of Energy's Brookhaven National Laboratory have found new clues to how the brain and the stomach interact with emotions to cause overeating, obesity and other mood-related behaviours.

Nutrition affects the brain in three ways:

1. **Brain cells** need proper nutrition to carry on their functions just like any other cell in the body.

2. The **myelin sheath** covering the brain cell acts like insulation covering electrical wires. It speeds transmission of electrical signals to the brain. Deficiencies in nutrition delay nerve-impulse transmission, negatively impacting brain function.

3. Some of the nutrients in the food we eat affect the **neurotransmitters**, such as serotonin, dopamine and norepinephrine, which carry messages from one cell to another and affect mood as well as thoughts and actions.

Below are foods that impact the brain positively or negatively:

Brain builders

Avocados, bananas, brewers' yeast, broccoli, brown rice, Brussels sprouts, cantaloupe, flaxseed oil, greens, legumes, oatmeal, oranges, peas, potatoes, romaine lettuce, soybeans, spinach, walnuts, wheat germ

Brain drainers

Alcohol, artificial food colourings, artificial sweeteners, colas, corn syrup, frostings, high-sugar drinks, hydrogenated fats, junk sugars, nicotine, overeating, white bread

Nutritional specifics

The essential for sustaining good brain function and peak performance is to ensure that you have an adequate intake of water and the correct proportion of proteins, carbohydrates, fats, vitamins and minerals. A good example of this can be acquired using the vegetarian food pyramid advocated by the General Conference Health department.*

Proteins

The amino acids from the breakdown of protein in the body are essential for building neurotransmitters – the brain's 'messengers'.

Vegetarians, and vegans in particular, need to consume the right combinations of foods to ensure they are getting the essential amino acids. Complete protein combinations, for example, are:

• Legumes (beans, chickpeas) or fresh vegetables combined with grains, pasta or brown rice. Dishes like maize and beans, tortillas and chickpeas, and dhal and chapattis are good combinations.

• Lentils or beans with mixed nuts.

• Sesame seeds or Brazil nuts with fresh vegetables.

Carbohydrates

When carbohydrate foods are
digested, glucose is released into the
bloodstream. This is vital to fuel the
brain and provide energy.
Carbohydrates fall into two categories:
slow-releasing or complex
carbohydrates and fast-releasing or
refined carbohydrates.

Slow-releasing carbohydrates:

• Brown rice, wholegrain pasta, dark
rye bread, fresh fruits and vegetables

These foods are high in fibre which
helps to slow down the release
of blood sugar.

Fast-releasing carbohydrates:

- Sweets, honey, sugary/processed cereals and white bread

These refined foods break down into glucose quickly and flood the body with too much sugar. This causes the brain to receive an energy surge, followed by a dramatic drop in glucose which results in decreased energy, shorter attention span and lack of concentration.

Try the following tips to maintain an even supply of glucose to the brain:

- Always have breakfast – include porridge oats, wholegrain cereal and bread instead of refined and sugary cereals.

- Avoid sugars and sweets.

- Avoid white flour, white rice.

- Avoid caffeine in coffee, tea and cola drinks.

- Omit alcohol.
- Eat slow-releasing carbohydrates and small amounts of protein if you combine them at mealtimes.
- Reduce stress.
- Exercise regularly.

* You can order a copy of the Vegetarian Food Pyramid by calling +1-301-680-6717.

The food pyramid for vegans can be found at *www.veganfoodpyramid.com*.

Eat the right fats

Now we take a closer look at 'healthy' and 'unhealthy' fats and their impact on brain health.

The three types of fat found in our foods are: saturated (mainly from animal products and junk foods), monounsaturated and polyunsaturated fats.

Saturated fats are known to increase the risk of atherosclerosis (fatty deposits or plaque) which blocks the blood vessels in the brain, negatively affecting brain function.

'Good fats' or 'essential fatty acids' are two specific fats called omega-3 and omega-6 (polyunsaturated fats). Studies indicate that these fats can increase the number of brain cells, enlarge the brain and improve learning and brain function.

Omega-3 and brain nutrition

Medical studies have shown that omega-3 oils play an important role in brain development. Strong evidence also supports the fact that omega-3 fatty acids can help with the development of the nervous system and the reduction of blood cholesterol.

Foods rich in omega-3

• The richest sources of omega-3 are algae, oily fish, broccoli, walnuts and flaxseed (ground/milled flaxseed or flaxseed oil are best). Flax oil is also available in vegetable capsules.

• Other sources of omega-3 are: olive oil, leafy green vegetables, pumpkin seeds and soya beans.

Some recent news reports indicate that there could be health risks associated with eating too much oily fish, in particular, salmon. This is because oily fish contains pollutants called dioxins and also PCBs (polychlorinated biphenyls), known to be toxic to humans.

A safer way to get sufficient omega-3
is to try alternating the food sources
in the chart below.

Good sources of omega-3 fats

Flaxseed oil	1 tablespoon (14g)
Flaxseed, ground	1 tablespoon (24g)
Rape seed oil	1 tablespoon (14g)
Walnuts	1oz (28g)
Tofu	4.5oz (126g)

Advice

- Eat more walnuts and broccoli.

- Include 4 to 5 teaspoons of ground flaxseeds, or rape seed oil in your diet.

- Do not heat these oils, as heating will alter the fat composition and reduce its efficacy.

- Add flaxseeds to foods just before serving. It is important that the flaxseeds are ground or at least crushed, as it makes the fat more readily available.

Nervous system nutrients

The central nervous system consists of the brain, the spinal cord and a large network of nerves throughout the body. The brain uses the information it receives from the nerves to co-ordinate all actions and reactions. A key vitamin crucial to brain health is Vitamin B.

B vitamins

- Help the body release energy from food to support vitality and stamina.

- Also help the nervous system carry information to and from the brain.

- Vitamin B12 in particular is essential for cell growth and replication and helps to support nerve and brain health.

- The anti-stress vitamin pantothenic acid (vitamin B5) is essential for normal physiological functions.

Vegetarian sources of vitamin B

Vitamin	Source
B1 (thiamine)	Soya beans, brown rice, sunflower seeds
B2 (riboflavin)	Almonds, mushrooms, whole grains
B3 (niacin)	Legumes, whole grains, avocado
B5 (pantothenic acid)	Brewers' yeast, mushrooms, avocado, egg yolk, whole grains
B6 (pyridoxine)	Whole grains, legumes, bananas, seeds, nuts
B12[1] (cobalamine)	Eggs, fortified soya cheese
Folic acid	Leafy green vegetables, legumes, nuts, eggs, wheat germ
Biotin	Nuts, brewers' yeast, egg yolk
Choline	Nuts, pulses, citrus fruits, wheat germ, egg yolk

[1]Vegans are recommended to eat foods fortified with vitamin B12 – yeast extracts, Vecon vegetable stock, veggie burger mixes, soya products, vegetable and sunflower margarines and breakfast cereals.

Vitamin D

New studies on vitamin D suggest that it may help promote brain health. Once vitamin D is converted in the body to its active form, calcitriol, it binds to receptors in the brain.

Sources: The main source of vitamin D is from sunlight on our skin. Other sources include eggs and dairy products and fortified foods. Vegans require vitamin D from fortified foods such as cereals, soya milk and margarine or supplements, particularly in winter.

Minerals

Magnesium works with B vitamins to help the body release energy from food and enhance nervous system and muscle function.

Sources: Cashews, beetroot, dates, raisins and soya beans.

Zinc – the brain's antioxidant. Also protects the blood brain barrier against toxins.

Sources: Beans, lentils, peanuts, seeds, wholegrain cereals.

Foods and the nervous system

Research is increasingly demonstrating that the brain is dependent on adequate supplies of nutrients in order to function properly. However, studies also show that when the brain does not receive these nutrients a number of deficiencies are exhibited. This produces a variety of negative symptoms affecting thought patterns, mood, emotion, perception and behaviour.

Considerable scientific data is emerging that links artificial stimulants and food additive intolerance to various mental and physical disorders.

Scientific evidence now supports a more natural diet for the enhancement of brain health and the avoidance of sugary and artificial foods.

In a recent article, 'Food for the Brain' the following breakfast menu was advocated for brain boosting:

Porridge oats with 1 tablespoon ground seeds (flax/linseeds, sesame, pumpkin, sunflower) Chopped fresh fruit or a spoonful of sugar-free jam (Add ground cinnamon or ginger for extra flavour if desired) Sugar-free cornflakes such as those by Doves Farm or Evernat.

There are specific foods which have been found to enhance brain function, invigorate the nervous system, as well as having a calming effect on the nerves. Below are a variety of symptoms/disorders and the associated foods that impact them.

Nervousness/anxiety

Increase: Oats, wheat germ, whole grains, Brazil nuts, walnuts, cashews, bananas, sunflower seeds

Avoid: Alcohol, stimulant beverages, meat, white sugar

Depression

Increase: Almonds, chickpeas, Brazil nuts, cashews, pine nuts, avocado, brewers' yeast, oats, wheat germ

Avoid: Saturated fats, stimulant beverages, alcoholic beverages, white sugar

Stress

Increase: Almond, chickpeas, pine nuts, oats, walnut, wheat germ,

Avoid: Stimulant beverages, alcoholic beverages, white sugar

Alzheimer's disease

Increase: Leafy green vegetables, brewers' yeast, wheat germ

Avoid: Cured cheeses, alcoholic beverages, stimulant drinks

Check your intake of these foods over the next month and if you need to make changes note any significant improvement in your mental wellbeing.

Eating patterns and brain health

Overeating

A report by Robert Preidt examines research from Texas Southwestern Medical Centre which suggests that overeating, not obesity, may be the actual cause of metabolic syndrome. The term metabolic syndrome refers to a group of health factors that increase the risk of developing insulin resistance, type 2 diabetes, heart disease and fatty liver. All these factors negatively impact brain health.

Food and mood

Current findings from scientists reveal that compulsive eating is regulated by the emotional centre in the brain, leading some people to overeat in an attempt to feel better. The desire to overeat (particularly in obese people) is controlled by the same part of the brain that controls cravings for drugs in addicts.

Gene-Jack Wang from the Centre for Translational Neuroimaging at Brookhaven National Laboratory, New York, states: 'We were able to simulate the process that takes place when the stomach is full, and for the first time we could see the pathway from the stomach to the brain that turns "off" the brain's desire to continue eating.' (Alok Jha, *The Guardian*, 3 October 2006.)

Brain chemistry

Low brain serotonin levels increase the temptation to reach for foods and substances which provide a temporary boost – sugary foods, refined carbohydrates (such as crisps, white bread and other processed foods) and alcohol. These foods perpetuate the cycle of cravings.

Advice

• A mostly plant-based diet helps keep serotonin and blood sugar stable and avoids snacking and overeating.

• Eat a good breakfast to avoid hypoglycaemia (low blood sugar) which can result in nervousness, irritability and low mood.

• Eat at regular times to avoid a sharp drop in blood glucose impacting brain nutrition and oxygenation.

Dietary practice impacting wellbeing

Current research suggests that Alzheimer's disease, like heart disease and strokes, is linked to the saturated fat, cholesterol and toxins found in meat and dairy products.

Recently the World Alzheimer's Congress reported on a large study which found that meat eaters had a higher risk of Alzheimer's. Conversely, people who remained free from any form of dementia had consumed higher amounts of vegetables, beta-carotene, vitamin C and vitamin E than people in the study who had developed Alzheimer's disease and had significant meat consumption.

The investigators found a strong correlation between increased cholesterol levels and increases in the number of plaques and tangles in the brain – two key elements of Alzheimer's disease. In contrast, the protective properties of plants, including antioxidants, vitamins and minerals, helped to lower the risk of developing Alzheimer's substantially and promoted overall good health.

Coffee's well-documented side effects have a list that includes anxiety, insomnia, tremor, irregular heartbeat, irritated bladder, prostate and digestive system.

Professor Chris Idzikowski, director of the Sleep Assessment Advisory Service in London, reports that high doses of strong coffee can slow down the metabolism so severely, the caffeine can stay in the body for up to 15 hours, affecting sleep. The stimulant effect of caffeine also interrupts the flow of melatonin, the brain hormone that induces sleep.

Emotional impact

Here we explore the emotional aspects of brain health. We include internal stimuli such as thought patterns and brain chemistry and external influences such as social influences and environmental factors. Also examined is the role of trauma and certain medications in relation to emotional wellness. Food and mood will also be analysed in relation to the nutritional impact on emotional wellbeing.

Brain chemistry

Science is currently able to assess the biological effects of the nervous system and chemical elements associated with emotional wellness. One such area examined is that of anxiety disorders. Researchers at The University of Manchester's Faculty of Medical and Health Sciences are studying the relationship between the biology of the nervous system, anxiety symptoms and behavioural problems.

In particular, they have progressed studies in the area of a condition called *generalised anxiety disorder* (GAD) which relates to excessive worrying. Anxiety disorders like GAD are due to changes in the activity of the brain circuits which deal with anxiety. The research indicates that abnormalities in brain serotonin (the neurotransmitter which regulates mood, emotion, sleep and appetite) influence these emotion circuits.

Mood and food

The nutritional aspect of food has also been found to affect mood. For example, a UK study by Benton and Cook (providing similar results to several other studies) demonstrates an association between low selenium intake and a significantly greater incidence of depression and other negative mood states. Additionally, several studies report changes in eating patterns when individuals are stressed.

Mental wellbeing

Mental health encompasses the emotional, spiritual and social resilience which enables us to achieve our full potential, to enjoy life, and to have the flexibility to deal with life's challenges, disappointments and sadness.

Scientific evidence increasingly points to the importance of building emotional wellbeing. Engaging individuals in activities designed to build self-esteem, coping skills and social support, benefits both individuals and communities. This is demonstrated in terms of emotional stability, positive physical health, enhanced social wellbeing and improved community cohesion.

Our minds are intricately connected to all aspects of our wellbeing. The field of psychosomatic disorders (which looks at the mind-body relationship and resulting illnesses) highlights the state of mind affecting the health of the body and vice versa. Additionally, our personal relationships and work abilities are affected by both mental health and physical issues.

The following examples are useful for assessing your wellbeing.

Emotions: Do you have a general sense of wellbeing and contentment?

Attitudes: Do you have the resilience to deal with life's stresses and bounce back from adversity? Do you have the ability to enjoy life, to laugh and have fun?

Life balance: Do you have a sense of balance in your life – between work and leisure, solitude and sociability, sleep and wakefulness, rest and exercise? Do you see yourself as well rounded – giving equal attention to mind, body, spirit?

Relationships: How easily do you care for yourself and others and enjoy positive relationships?

Prospective thinking: Do you look at the future with hope?

Self-realisation: Are you able to participate in life to the best of your ability, engaging in meaningful activities, pursuing your full potential?

Adaptability: How flexible are you to life's changing circumstances? Do you have the ability to adapt, grow and cope with a range of feelings that accompany change?

We deal with varying feelings and emotions on a daily basis. Sometimes these are fairly easy to cope with and sometimes they become challenging.

Factors influencing emotional wellbeing

Mental health challenges are usually the outcome of the varying experiences in a person's life, from early childhood to later life events. Various contributory factors are considered when analysing the development of most mental health problems.

The following categories give an outline of causes and risk factors associated with mental and emotional health challenges.

Sociological/environmental

Serious early life losses or traumas – death of a parent in childhood, abuse, neglect, severe injury, war experiences.

Loss of social support – death of a loved one, divorce, estranged/moved away from family/friends, loss of job, loss of trust.

Chaotic, unsafe or dangerous environments – violent home, homelessness, abject poverty.

Physiological

Genetic causes – close family history of depression.

Chronic illness – dependent on medication and/or illnesses seriously restricting activity.

Hormonal changes – menstrual cycle changes and life stage adjustments that affect mood.

Biological causes – imbalanced neurotransmitters like decreased serotonin, known to affect thought processes and emotions.

Medical

Medication side effects – drugs used for chronic illnesses.

Experiential

Negative experiences that undermine self-confidence – work-related or relationship failures.

Negative thought patterns and learned helplessness – repeated or chronic stressful events resulting in feelings of helplessness, reinforced by lack of control over the situation.

Experiential

Substance abuse – depressive effects can results from use of alcohol and drugs. Additionally, the negative personal and social consequences of substance abuse can also be a contributing factor to depression. It is still unclear, however, which comes first – attempting to control depression with substances, or the use of substances that then cause depression.

Tips for promoting good emotional and mental health

• List the things that are troubling you.

• Prioritise your challenges on that list and deal with the simplest ones or the most stressful issue that you can give your immediate attention to.

• Get adequate rest.

• Eat a balanced diet.

• Avoid caffeine, alcohol, tobacco, or other drugs.

• Engage in physical activities.

- Nurture your spiritual needs by prayer and reflection time with God.

- Appreciate the beauty in nature.

- Spend adequate time with people whose company you enjoy or those who are positive and upbeat.

- Undertake a fun or relaxing activity – go for scenic walks, listen to music, read a good book, watch a humorous video, talk to a friend and so on.

Mental activity and brain function

It is evident that our social experiences, personal relationships and work abilities interrelate with our physical and mental health issues. During times of intense stress, when we are distressed or experience great anxiety, our physical health can be affected and we can feel emotionally low.

Mental activity and the brain

Research in the field of neurological brain function and stimulation demonstrates a link with memory and mood. The phrase 'use it or lose it' in this context is certainly most pertinent to individuals who begin to notice a decline in their abilities to retain and process information, particularly with advancing age.

Mental stimulation may have a preventative effect on illnesses such as dementia and Alzheimer's disease. One US study asked subjects to review their 20s, 30s, 40s and 50s and report on their regular leisure activities. Researchers found that people who had undertaken more intellectual activities in their 20s and 30s had a lower risk of developing Alzheimer's. The activities included doing jigsaws and other puzzles, playing a musical instrument, doing crafts or home repairs, playing board games, writing letters, reading. Subjects demonstrating increased intellectual activities after their 30s had a reduced Alzheimer's risk of up to 47%.

Key research finding: Engaging in stimulating brain activity may assist in creating increased cognitive reserve, enhancing brain adaptability and compensating for other damaged areas.

Advice: The brain is a muscle that requires exercise as do other body muscles.

Tips for daily mental stimulation

Over the next two weeks, try the following suggestions below and observe the difference it makes to your mental alertness and mood.

- Engage in a crossword, jigsaw or other puzzles

- Step up your practice if you play a musical instrument

- Commence a creative activity or re-engage in a favourite craft that you've neglected

- Tackle a household repair that you have been putting off for some time

- Play board games

- Write a letter to a friend or family member

- Complete a book in the next two weeks

Emotions and mental activity

Richard J. Davidson of the Laboratory for Functional Brain Research at the Institute of Wisconsin-Madison revealed MRI scan (magnetic resonance imaging) results which identified the relationship between brain activity and emotional states. He found a distinctive difference between the brains of individuals characterised by enthusiasm, alertness, energy, persistence in goal orientation and other positive behavioural characteristics in comparison with the brains of those individuals who experienced depression.

From his research a possible link has been found between the functioning of a region of the brain called the *amygdale*, responsible for processing emotions. 'We've already discovered that there are differences in the *amygdales* of people who appear to be happy, positive individuals compared with those of individuals who show more vulnerability and more depressive emotion in response to the emotional events in life,' he states.

It was found that the right frontal area of that region was more active when negative emotions and stress were experienced. In contrast Davidson noted that the left side was activated when positive emotions were expressed. He also stated, 'In infancy and early childhood, individuals with the pattern of left prefrontal activity show signs of exuberance and are highly social.'

Psychology researcher Kalin comments: 'Scientists have begun to redirect their attention from problems that produce disease to brain systems that regulate positive emotions and their relationship to key physiological systems affecting health.'

The Cleveland Clinic Foundation highlights research on the following activities which stimulate brain activity and enhance emotional wellbeing:

- **Prayer** – Brain imaging studies show that brain activity changes during prayer. Research indicates that blood pressure and heart rate can decrease during times of prayer.

- **Music therapy** – Particularly in clinical settings, the therapeutic effects of music in relieving pain and reducing stress and anxiety have been extensively researched.

- **Massage** – Patients experiencing anxiety can receive beneficial short-term effects. Massage has been found to improve relaxation, relieve muscle tension, improve sleep and enhance blood circulation.

Emotional wellness – the stress and trauma impact

We all experience emotional pain at some point in our lives and stressful moments are common to most of us. However, persistent stress, mental fatigue and anger affect our mood and behaviour and, ultimately, our outlook on life.

Medical research demonstrates the connection between long-standing stress and holistic wear and tear. The consequence of poor response to stress and trauma not only has emotional effects but also has a negative physical impact.

Studies show the chemical changes that take place in the brain when we process negative thoughts. Neurological tests also demonstrate the energy drain that occurs in the body, affecting muscle response, co-ordination and reaction time. Science concludes that the more negative emotion becomes part of our daily life, it leads to premature damage of our cells. Stress, feeling out of control, anger, fear, grief, sadness and depression all have a negative effect on our cells and immune system, leading to further disease. (The neurobiology of stress, 2000.)

With effective stress management, social and lifestyle changes can usually restore physiological and psychological balance. This is not necessarily the case when someone becomes traumatised. 'Traumatisation is stress frozen in place – locked into a pattern of neurological distress that doesn't go away by returning to a state of equilibrium.' (*HealingResources.info*) This requires professional intervention.

Fact:

- Positive thoughts create positive feelings which motivate positive actions.

- Positive beliefs influence our whole approach to life.

- Our feelings, thoughts and beliefs can be changed from negative to positive.

- Traumatic life events can be difficult to deal with. Individuals in these situations require support (sometimes professional help) to enable them to deal with the memories, find positive coping mechanisms and move forward with their life.

Exercise:

- Identify your feelings, thoughts and beliefs and how they impact your response to life events.

- Instead of believing that you always fail at tasks, try stating that you do the best you can with the help of God.

- If you see yourself as being helpless in any given situation, realise that you can take control and that God is ultimately in charge.

Chemical and hormonal impact

Brain response to body chemicals and stress hormones

With increasing scientific insight into the consequences of stress on the brain, the picture that emerges is a sobering one. Chronic overreaction to stress overloads the brain with powerful hormones only intended for short-term work in emergency situations. The cumulative effect of continuous stress impairs the brain's ability to learn and remember new information. It also damages and even kills brain cells. This is because the continuous over-secretion of stress hormones like cortisol adversely affects brain function and memory.

Brain response to stress

• The key brain area dealing with stress is called the limbic system. It is frequently referred to as 'the emotional brain' because of its enormous influence on emotions and memory.

• Renowned brain researcher Robert M. Sapolsky reports that sustained stress can damage a part of the limbic brain – the hippocampus which is central to learning and memory.

• Corticosteroids (cortisol) and adrenaline are secreted from the adrenal glands during stress. Once in the brain, cortisol remains much longer than adrenalin where it continues to affect brain cells.

Memory formation and retrieval

- During a stressful situation we sometimes forget important information. This is because cortisol interferes with the function of neurotransmitters, the chemicals that brain cells use to communicate with each other.

- Excessive cortisol can affect thinking ability and retrieval of long-term memories.

Memory loss

• Stress hormones divert blood glucose to key muscles, which reduces the amount of glucose (energy) reaching the brain's hippocampus. This results in an energy crisis in the hippocampus, compromising its ability to create new memories.

• In his book *Brain Longevity*, Dharma Singh Khalsa MD identifies some older people losing 20-25% of their hippocampus cells. This causes short-term memory which is a feature of age-related memory loss resulting from a lifetime of stress.

Cortisol and brain degeneration

• Mayo Clinic researchers using magnetic resonance imaging found that specific hippocampus changes were linked to altered behaviour associated with ageing and Alzheimer's disease.

• Neurologist Ronald C. Petersen, principal author of the study, states: 'When certain parts of the hippocampus shrink or deteriorate, specific, related memory abilities are affected.' Hippocampus size averaged 14% smaller in the group showing high and rising cortisol levels, compared to the group with moderate and decreasing levels. The small hippocampus group also did worse at memory tests and pictures they'd seen 24 hours earlier.

Environmental factors

Ongoing studies continue to demonstrate that certain environmental agents can interfere with specific stages of brain development, interrupt brain cell division, alter gene expression, differentiate into specialised cell types, establish connections with other brain cells, interfere with chemical messengers in the brain that help transmit nerve impulses and cause brain cell death.

Following is a list of chemical pollutants that negatively impact brain health.

Alcohol crosses the placenta and affects varying stages of brain development. The exposed foetus may develop into a child with hyperactivity, learning challenges, lowered IQ or, in severe cases, mental retardation.

Aluminium. Overexposure to aluminium compounds – in cookware, foil, antacids, deodorants and toothpaste – can adversely affect brain function.

Bisphenol A (chemical found in many plastic containers) can alter the expression of genes required for early brain development and long-term memory formation.

Lead. Exposure in childhood may lead to attention problems, hyperactivity, impulsive behaviour, reduced IQ, poor school performance, aggression and delinquent behaviour.

Manganese. Elevated levels are associated with ADHD, hyperactivity and Parkinson's disease.

Mercury crosses the placenta and can affect brain development, IQ, language development, visual-spatial skills, memory and attention span.

Polychlorinated biphenyls (PCBs) are industrial chemicals which, although banned, still linger in the environment. They have been identified in the body's fatty tissue and can impair reflexes, IQ, delay mental and motor skills development and cause hyperactivity.

Solvents like toluene cause learning, speech and motor skill challenges in children. These effects were discovered in studies of children whose mothers sniffed glue during pregnancy.

Tobacco smoke/nicotine. Much research reveals their toxicity, particularly to the developing brain. Smoking during pregnancy affects the mental development of the child later on, putting them more at risk for learning disorders, lower IQ and attention deficits. Passive smoking is also a risk. Children born to women who are passively exposed to cigarette smoke have higher levels of impaired speech, poor language skills and lower intelligence. Additionally, children exposed to tobacco smoke following birth are also at risk for various behavioural problems.

Prions are an infectious form of a protein type, thought to be the agents responsible for the rare brain disorder variant Creutzfeldt-Jakob Disease (CJD) in humans and mad cow disease. People can be exposed to prions by eating contaminated food or other products made from animals with diseases such as mad cow disease.

Be vigilant!

Improving brain function

Brain training, memory enhancement and the improvement of brain efficacy are topical areas of research. Keeping the brain fit, particularly as we age, is well researched in its positive impact on emotional and mental wellbeing as well as guarding against age-related illnesses such as dementia and Alzheimer's disease. Several publications now boast the solution to optimum brain enhancement.

An issue of the magazine *Puzzler Brain Trainer* lists in its contents: mind-toning workouts; memory jog exercises; live and learn – how learning can keep you young; brain box and a number of other intriguing activities aimed at maximising brain stimulation. The author, Ian Robertson, is a neuroscientist, trained clinical psychologist and leading world expert on neuropsychology relating to brain rehabilitation. The brain teasers, exercises and tips in the magazine challenge the reader to use his brain to its full potential. I encourage you to take part in similar mental challenges to test the theories of brain improvement.

The book *Use It or Lose It* by Allen D. Bragdon and David Gamon of the Brainwaves Center, is based on recent research in the area of neurosciences. It is a useful resource which offers readers mental acuity tests, mind maintenance techniques and exercises that build mental skills.

It has been stated that individuals learn best when their experience is not just theoretical but incorporates more practical, inspirational and fun aspects.

Enhancing mental capacity

Neuroscientists are discovering how flexible the brain is. It was once thought that the adult brain only lost cells (neurones) and was not able to replace them. Current research reveals that the new neurones and the connections between them continue to develop throughout life well into the senior years. This process of acquiring new brain cells is called neuroplasty, and research now shows that it can be harnessed to help protect and enhance our mental capacity.

Science is proving that the brain responds to mental stimulation much like a muscle responding to physical exercise. So, just as we give the body regular workouts to enhance health and wellbeing, in the same way the brain requires regular workouts to enhance its efficacy.

Facts:

• The more diverse and vigorous your mental activity, the more you are able to handle mental challenges.

• The greater the mental fitness, the more you will stimulate the growth of new neurones and new connections between them.

• The type of mental activity you undertake determines in which area of the brain growth takes place.

These facts were discovered by combining experiments from real-life situations and the use of high-resolution technologies (neuroimaging), particularly MRI brain scans. Studies revealed that certain parts of the brain were larger in individuals who used that section of the brain more than most people.

Research findings:

• The part of the brain critical for spatial memory – the hippocampus – was larger than usual in London cab drivers, who generally have to navigate and remember complex routes in large city areas.

• A part of the temporal lobe of the brain – Heschl's gyrus – involved in processing music, is larger in professional musicians than in non-musical individuals.

• The part of the brain involved in language – the Angular gyrus – proved to be larger in bilingual individuals than those only speaking one language.

Evaluation: The extent to which a specific area of the brain was enlarged was directly related to the amount of time the individual spent on activities stimulating that brain area. So the hippocampal size was larger in brains of cab drivers the more years they spent on the job, and the size of Heschl's gyrus related to the amount of time musicians devoted to practising their musical instrument.

Tip: Increase mental activity to increase brain capacity.

Stimulation and learning

Ten essential brain boosters
for learning:

1. As physical exercise keeps the body fit, so mental exercise enhances brain activity. If you don't exercise it, like your body, the brain will become 'flabby'. We strengthen our mental muscles and brain capacity by challenging them.

2. Attempt a new skill like learning to play a musical instrument. This boosts brain activity and stimulates brain cells and capacity, regardless of age.

3. Three key elements to good learning are: challenge, change and new information. Activities that involve an element of challenge that becomes more difficult as you improve is best. The activity should include change which involves fresh situations and tasks as these switch on additional brain cells. Learning something new grows new brain connections, enhancing brain stimulation.

4. Brain-training games and exercises are fun ways to keep the brain active. Keep a puzzle book close at hand for brain-boosting moments.

5. Include other stimulating activities like meeting new people, reading, improving your cooking or learning a new language.

6. People (interesting ones) are a good stimulant. A rich network of friends boosts the brain and increases our connectivity and interaction with others.

7. Aerobic exercise is an excellent brain enhancer. Check with your GP what best suits you.

8. Stress and low mood can suppress brain function. Learning to manage these challenges is crucial for mental wellbeing.

9. Proper nutrition (particularly group B vitamins and omega-3) is crucial to maintaining brain health, as is adequate rest which rejuvenates the brain.

10. Memory enhancing activities are key to effective stimulation of the brain. Try to memorise something new every day as it keeps the brain sharp. Learning passages of Scripture is one beneficial exercise as it boosts both mental and spiritual health.

Learning and retention

Paced learning: Research demonstrates that people who 'cram' or 'speed learn' do not necessarily come away with as deep and permanent an understanding of the material as those who study at a more steady and regular pace. Gerald W. Bracey, an educational psychologist and associate professor at George Mason University, found that students who tried to learn large amounts in a short period of time did less well than students who studied the same volume of information over a longer time. When students were tested six months later, those who studied in a more in-depth fashion had retained more information that the 'crammers'.

Goal setting: When learning a new skill, set small goals which are achievable and undertake them in small steps rather than rushing to achieve the overall goal as quickly as possible. This will ensure that the learning is well grounded and that you take on manageable portions as you build steadily towards your goal. The brain retains new information better this way. Also as you compare your achievement with these small steps and do not expect to be able to grasp the new skill quickly, it is more likely that you will stay the course.

The sleep impact

A shocking headline appeared in *New Scientist* on 6 September 2003: 'Lack of sleep can cause brain damage and affect memory'. Sleep is important; but surely losing some sleep could not amount to so much damage, could it? In this fast-paced, pressurised world we sometimes find ourselves with too much to do and not enough time to accomplish it. In an attempt to meet deadlines and squeeze more into a twenty-four-hour period than is reasonably possible, we can find ourselves cutting back on much-needed sleep. Now scientists are finding that this is to our detriment.

Roxanne Khamsi, reporting in *New Scientist* on 11 February 2009, highlighted a new study which demonstrates that sleep deprivation can severely hamper the brain's ability to learn. In an experiment led by Seung-Schik Yoo and colleagues at Harvard Medical School in Boston, Massachusetts, US, the study demonstrated that people who failed to get a good night's sleep before studying new information did not retain as much information as individuals who slept well. In fact, the results showed that they remembered roughly 10% less than their well-rested counterparts.

The researchers concluded that it was 'a worrying finding', particularly in light of other current findings which suggested that the average amount of sleep people get each night is decreasing.

'This study shows that the brain has to be well rested to receive and store information for memory processing,' stated Seung-Schik Yoo. Previous studies have also shown that a full night's rest after studying can improve learning.

So what happens to the brain
during sleep?

Scientists have found that *when we're
asleep, our brain continues to learn the
material we've been exposed to while
we were awake*. From all the
information that the brain processed
during the day, it derives meaning.
Subconsciously the brain analyses the
information and works through
unsolved problems. During this
process the physical structure of the
brain cells alters so that specific
pieces of knowledge are etched more
permanently in memory. Neurologists
refer to this process as **consolidation**.

Facts

- Adequate sleep is essential for study, retention and retrieval of information.

- Hours of sleep gained before midnight are twice as valuable and restful to body and mind as the hours after midnight.

- An hour of work in the morning is twice as productive as an hour of work late at night.

Age-related brain maintenance

The following age-related activity has been found to be effective for brain maintenance.

0-10

Language is fundamental to cognitive development. Talking and listening to children is one of the best ways to make the most of their critical brain-building years. Children who engage in lots of verbal interaction show more advanced linguistic skills than children who don't.

From age 10 onwards The Brainwaves Center suggests the following to maintain mental capacity as we age.

10 plus

Working out why things happen, not just what is happening, is a great stimulant to the brain building new neural pathways.

20 plus

When reading an article, imagine that later you have to express your opinion to someone else on what you have learned through it. This stimulates neurons. Eighty percent of the neurons that activate when you do something physically are activated when you *imagine* doing it.

40s

Puzzles and games that require analysis of facts are great for challenging the brain. Another great brain-exercise technique that enhances short- and long-term memory is to concentrate closely on what another person is saying to you. This builds concentration ability.

50s

The brain shifts resources continually. For each task that it has to accomplish, the brain recruits circuits. Disused brain circuits inhibit this ability. So keep challenging your mind with tasks. Although some brain cells are lost over time, the remaining cells become effective when worked harder.

65 plus

The brain works best when there are multiple new things to learn. In later years, people are not compelled to learn new skills. This slows down brain capacity. Therefore attempting new challenges continually keeps the mind sharp.

Facts

• The latest brain boosting exercise, neurobics, enhances overall mental fitness and flexibility as we age. It challenges the brain with non-routine experiences to expand brain capacity.

• Neurobics involves doing things you normally do, but doing them differently. For example, writing or brushing your teeth with the opposite hand, taking a different route to work and so on.

• During these neurobic exercises the underused nerve pathways and connections in the brain become activated. This stimulates growth of new brain cells and brain connections.

Try alternating the above neurobic exercises on an ongoing basis.

The spiritual impact

At a 2009 nutrition conference Angelette Muller, Nutrition Consultant and University Lecturer in Nutritional Therapy, spoke about the link between diet, appetite, mind and spirituality. She highlighted the brain's pre-frontal cortex responsible for 'higher cognitive functions' which allows us to exercise self-control and decision-making and factors that affect it.

A recent article by Robin Nixon carried the title 'Spirituality spot found in the brain'. It was found that individuals who were more spiritual had physiological differences in the parietal lobe of their brain. Researcher Brick Johnstone of Missouri University also concluded that a positive spiritual outlook has been associated with better mental and physical health. Previous research on neuro-spirituality using brain scans of practising 'believers' resulted in broad and inconclusive findings, as it was not clear whether subjects were responding to their life experience or specific religious practice. However, in recent studies, researchers looked for correlations between brain region performance and the subjects' self-reported spirituality which demonstrated a significant link.

The psychological impact

What about hypnosis?

Research indicates that hypnosis may reduce activity in certain brain areas. Miranda Hitti, in an article entitled 'What Hypnosis Does to the Brain' (2005), discussed how a study at Cornell University's medical school had demonstrated the brain's sensitivity to hypnosis. The process appeared to lull brain areas into going along with suggestions made during hypnosis.

That theory was tested in a new study. Researchers used brain scans to watch the brain under the influence of hypnosis. Specialised MRI brain scans showed less activity in two areas of the hypnotised brain.

Sandra Blakeslee writes: 'Hypnosis, with its long and chequered history in medicine and entertainment, is receiving some new respect from neuroscientists. Recent brain studies of people who are susceptible to suggestion indicate that when they act on the suggestions their brains show profound changes in how they process information. The suggestions, researchers report, literally change what people see, hear, feel and believe to be true.'

She continues: 'The new experiments, which used brain imaging, found that people who were hypnotised "saw" colours where there were none. Others lost the ability to make simple decisions. Some people looked at common English words and thought that they were gibberish.'

Perception

Crucial to mental wellbeing is how we perceive the world around us.

• Our sensory organs receive signals which are then passed through the nervous system to the brain, which processes the information, whether from visual, auditory or tactile stimulation.

• Assisting the process are built-in filters which sift the information we take in. This, for example, would include how we deal with noise. We often filter out background noise so that we can concentrate on what we are doing without distraction.

• A bad experience, however, may become ingrained in the brain's 'programme'. If the individual is unable to filter the negative thoughts from that experience, it can affect how he/she rationalises that event or similar experiences.

• Attitudes and emotions can also affect the perception process. Scientific studies reveal our tendency to read the implications of another person's words and their body language differently, depending on how we feel about that individual.

• *Brain Research*, Volume 1079, Issue 1, 24 March 2006, details the link between perception and action and its impact on our decision-making process and social behaviour.

'. . . be transformed by the renewing of your mind.' Rom. 12:2.

Conclusion

'Use it or lose it' is true when it comes to brain health. The tips in this book are designed to enable you to utilise your grey matter to its full potential. Research has demonstrated the importance of keeping the brain active to preserve mental capacity. Equally important has been the undisputed evidence that highlights maintaining a healthy body as key to ensuring a healthy mind.

Educator Alvaro Fernandez lists what he calls the four pillars of brain health:

Mental exercise

Physical exercise

Nutrition

Stress management

Here is your list of 'must dos' for maintaining good brain health:

- Regularly play a variety of good brain games
- Eat brain healthy foods
- Ensure you undertake regular physical exercise
- Reduce stress
- Get adequate rest

- Detox your mind from a negative attitude
- Regularly make a list of all the things you are grateful for
- Try something new like taking a course or learning a new skill
- Learn a new language
- Spend more time with others to enhance social stimulation
- Nurture your prayer life and practise your faith

Good health to your brain!